LIVING
KIDNEY
STONES

LIVING WITH
KIDNEY
STONES

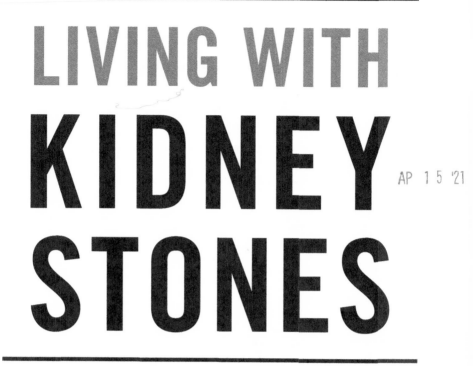

The Complete Guide to Risk Factors, Symptoms & Treatment Options

SAMANTHA BOWICK, MPH

Foreword by DAVID BRANDLI, MD

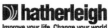

Improve your life. Change your world.

Hatherleigh Press is committed to preserving and protecting the natural resources of the earth. Environmentally responsible and sustainable practices are embraced within the company's mission statement.

Visit us at www.hatherleighpress.com and register online for free offers, discounts, special events, and more..

Living with Kidney Stones
Text copyright © 2021 Samantha Bowick

Library of Congress Cataloging-in-Publication Data is available upon request.
ISBN: 978-1-57826-886-3

Cover Design by Carolyn Kasper

Printed in the United States
10 9 8 7 6 5 4 3 2 1

DISCLAIMER: The authors of this book are not medical professionals and make no claims otherwise. The goal of this book is to provide patients and the public with information about kidney stones through one patient's story of living with the illness.

*For anyone who has ever suffered with the
excruciating pain of a kidney stone;
you are not alone.*

CONTENTS

FOREWORD BY DR. BRANDLI

A CROSS MEDICINE, the kidney stone patient is unique. While a symptomatic kidney stone is rarely life-threatening, it is one of the most painful experiences you can have on this earth. Along with the pain often follows nausea, vomiting, and a variety of urinary symptoms. And worse, kidney stones can be recurrent with patients having episodes often throughout their lives, with difficult episodes treated with pain medicines, antiemetics, and sometimes surgery.

With this also comes a unique opportunity for prevention. Kidney stones are largely preventable. And usually the prevention comes in the form of dietary changes and not medication, although medicines are sometimes beneficial.

Living with Kidney Stones examines the physiology, biochemistry, and genetics of kidney stones with an emphasis on understanding the interplay between these and the treatment avenues that this understanding provides. *Living with Kidney Stones* makes these principles accessible to all and gives an opportunity to avoid the painful recurrent cycles of stone attacks that make this condition so regrettable.

—David Brandli, MD

1

My Story

I 'D HAD kidney infections and urinary tract infections before, but I had never before experienced this type of sharp, persistent kidney pain. With urinary tract infections, I'd had pain when urinating, but I would take some antibiotics and the urinary tract infection would go away, at least for a little while. Then, after my excision surgery for endometriosis, I stopped getting urinary tract infections until the day after Christmas in 2018. To top it all off, I've suffered from nausea for the last decade off and on.

So when I felt nausea and some pain while urinating, I didn't really think much about it...until the horrible sharp pain on my right side sent me to the floor, forcing my parents to call an ambulance.

I know all about debilitating and gut-wrenching pain symptoms. Endometriosis, polycystic ovary syndrome, osteoporosis, irritable bowel syndrome, interstitial cystitis...my medical history is a laundry list of ailments that unfortunately get you pretty accustomed to pain. But this was a sort of unrelenting pain that came out of nowhere and wouldn't go away. Lying in bed and taking a hot bath didn't help; the pain was the same no matter which way I turned or laid. I didn't know what was going on or wrong with me. All I knew was that the pain occurred right after urinating early in the morning.

I had a small inkling it was a kidney stone only because my sister and brother had experienced them, but I could only hope I was wrong. I didn't have medical insurance to deal with something long-term or that could require multiple doctor appointments, procedures and tests, or surgery. And so it was that I arrived at the emergency room, conveniently located about twenty minutes from my home, where I would spend at least another 20 minutes sitting in the waiting room, wracked with agonizing pain.

The emergency medical technicians told me that, based on where my pain was located, they were sure it was a kidney stone. By this time, I had also started throwing up (my vomit was green, though I was told much later that this green color was because I do not have a gallbladder). But nausea and vomiting are not unique to kidney stones; it could still have been something else, I hoped. Which isn't to say I was thrilled about it: I couldn't remember the last time I had thrown up prior to this (though at a guess, it was likely four years prior when I had to do a bowel prep for endometriosis surgery).

A nurse saw me about 15 or 20 minutes later, though it took at least another hour and a half for a doctor to come in to see me. My mom tells me I was lying in the bed moaning, tossing, and turning and asking why nobody would help me at the time, which makes sense; I don't remember much about this emergency room trip myself, you see.

The doctor finally ordered a scan (mind you, I still hadn't received any pain or nausea medication even though I'd told them my symptoms when I arrived; even then, they could *see* that I was actively vomiting). I had to lie as still as I could for the scan to be completed accurately, which itself was extremely painful. It felt like I'd have to wait until after the scan results came back before anyone in the emergency room would believe my pain.

Finally, I received Toradol for the inflammation and pain and Zofran for the nausea. The Toradol relieved most of the pain I was experiencing within 20 minutes and the Zofran kept me from throwing up, which was a plus. I was then told that I had a three millimeter kidney stone on my right side and that I should be able to pass it on my own, which was more of a minus. In fact, I was terrified to try that because I'd heard the stories from my siblings, cousins, and others who have passed kidney stones. But no matter what happened, I knew I needed relief.

I was told to schedule an appointment with a urologist and discharged after being there a total of three hours. The next day, my mom called the urologist's office, only to learn that a doctor's referral was needed to be seen at all. Because the ER didn't send a referral to the local urologist, this meant if I had any more problems with the kidney stone, I would have to go back to the emergency room and risk getting sick, or my mom getting sick, all while paying a lot of money to be treated.

I'd been to see a urologist in the past to determine if my endometriosis pain and symptoms were urology related, but the one I went to before was not close to where I lived, so I needed to find a new one. My previous urologist told me to keep a diary of how much fluid I drank each day, and to measure my urine output to determine if I was urinating adequately. I also had to do a urine test in the office that measured my urine stream. I was told that all my test results were normal, but the urologist ordered an abdominal scan to be certain. He told me my results there were normal, too; it wasn't until I received an email later on from the online patient portal that I discovered the test actually showed I had free fluid in my pelvis, which had never even been mentioned by the doctor. It's so frustrating to have doctors not tell you your entire results, and it's happened to me enough times over the years to make me trust doctors less and rely on myself more. With that being said, there are amazing doctors out there who will go above and beyond for their patients; I don't want to discourage anyone from seeking medical care. I mention this only to illustrate the importance of taking an active role in your own health and healthcare—because nobody is going to care more about healing your body than you.

Exactly a week after my first visit, I was right back in the emergency room, writhing in pain and complaining of trouble urinating. I was drinking plenty of water, I just wasn't urinating as much as I was drinking. (At least this time I didn't need to go by ambulance!)

I arrived around 10 PM with my mother in tow. They took me straight to triage to check my temperature, blood pressure, and oxygen saturation level. I was told they were running behind (which didn't really surprise me, given that it was actually New Year's Eve) and that I would need to wait in the waiting room.

As the night progressed, my pain worsened. A couple of hours went by and nobody had been called back, so my mom went up to the front desk and asked what was going on. They told her they didn't have any rooms available yet; there were even patients being seen in the hall. Finally, I had my blood drawn and gave a urine sample and was told that, based on my results, I would need to be in a room.

After *ten* hours, I was finally called into a room. I was in immense pain by this point, but couldn't get any medication until a doctor saw me. If my pain hadn't worsened, I would have left by this point. I was also worried about my mom getting sick from being there because she has a weaker immune system.

Eventually, a doctor appeared. Another scan was ordered and I received Toradol for the pain and Zofran for nausea. (I wasn't throwing up, but felt like I could at any moment.) I was told that there was blood in my urine and that I was showing signs of infection, so I was given an antibiotic. I was also asked whether or not I wanted to have the scan done, given the risk posed by the radiation having just had a scan a week prior. It made me feel stupid, but I trusted my gut. I explained that I wanted the scan done because I was in so much pain.

The scan showed my kidney stone had not moved in a week, so the emergency room doctor tried to schedule an appointment for me with a urologist and wrote me a prescription for Zofran, Norco, an antibiotic, and Flomax (to help increase urination). When I was discharged, I was told to call the urologist's office on their next open day, because the ER hadn't been able to make the appointment for me. As this was New Year's, it took another two days before I was able to get ahold of anyone…only to be told that I'd missed my appointment window, despite having called first thing in the morning, as soon as they opened. Fortunately, they were able to work me in a couple of hours later.

Believe me when I say that I know how hard it is to advocate for yourself, especially when you are in a lot of pain and feel awful, but nobody knows how you feel as well as you. We know what we need and it's important that we get that point across when going to doctor appointments, the emergency room, etc.

To prove that point: after the second time I went to the emergency room, I logged in to take another look at my test results, only to find out that my liver enzymes were extremely elevated. The doctor had failed to discuss this with me at all, or even make me aware of it. To make matters worse, I'd had a complete blood panel done both times I went to the emergency room, which gave me a benchmark for comparison. The first time I went, my blood work was normal. The second time, my blood work wasn't normal. My liver tests were extremely abnormal and should have been discussed with me. Specifically, my ALT (alanine aminotransferase) was 691 (the normal range is 13–61), my AST level (aspartate aminotransferase) was

179 (the normal range is 15-37), and my ALK PHOS (alkaline phosphatase) level was 142 (the normal range is 45-117). All of these are indicators of liver complications.

My internal medicine doctor was not at all happy with how my case had been handled. She at least was very concerned about my test results, especially because I'm an alpha-1 anti-trypsin deficiency carrier. She ordered liver enzyme tests to be drawn the same day I visited, with a follow-up appointment one week later to go over the results.

The next week when I went back, my liver enzymes were mostly normal. Because I had never had problems with my liver (aside from a lesion back in 2016), we decided to chalk it up to pain medications, as I was taking Aleve and/or pre-scription Norco for my kidney stone pain interchangeably. (Though, after receiving these results, I stopped taking Norco for fear of it causing problems with my liver.) For the last ten years, I'd been taking pain medication on and off because of the chronic pain I have suffered related to endometriosis and other chronic illnesses, as well as for surgery recovery. I began to wonder if this had affected my liver in a negative way, given that many pain medications contain acetaminophen (Tylenol), which is metabolized in the liver, and why there are regulations on how much should be taken daily.

I went over my kidney stone symptoms with my urologist, and he said that while we could do surgery, it might be better if I waited and tried to pass the stone on my own. Left with no other realistic option, I agreed. By that point, I had been put under anesthesia at least 12 times in my life and I wanted to avoid seeing that number creep any higher. The doctor also told me to continue taking Flomax and said Azo was okay to continue taking, too. I scheduled a follow-up appointment with him for two weeks later and continued working in pain while taking Aleve to mitigate my symptoms as best I could.

After seeing the urologist, I needed to determine my best options. I was working as a pharmacy technician at the time, 2–4 hours three days a week; I was also working as a marketing coordinator from home for up to 10 hours each week. I *did* have the option of obtaining health insurance, but even then I still couldn't pay the premiums. (It wouldn't be until later on that I would discover I was still on Medicaid; however, that wouldn't have covered anything that I needed for my kidney stone.) I was fortunate that I'd not had to go to the doctor the previous year, something which hadn't occurred in the last ten years. All I could do was hope that the doctor was right, and that the stone would pass naturally.

During this time, I was overwhelmingly exhausted. Fatigue hit me hard; I spent most of my time lying in my bed, especially if I wasn't working. Pain drained me of my energy, making it hard to focus or do everyday tasks. This type of pain would leave anyone unable to go to work or school, instead relying on others to help in many ways.

By my next appointment, I was still in pain and was certain I hadn't passed the kidney stone. My urologist again gave me the option of having surgery, and as much as I *really* didn't want to have another surgery, I scheduled a lithotripsy for the following week. I just couldn't continue living in the amount of pain and nausea I was in, unable to function the way I needed to.

2

What Are Kidney Stones?

A CCORDING TO the National Kidney Foundation: "Each year, more than half a million people go to emergency rooms for kidney stones".[1] Added to that, about 1 out of every 10 people will experience a kidney stone sometime in their life—meaning kidney stones are more prevalent than COPD and about as prevalent as diabetes.

But what are kidney stones?

Before answering that, we first need to understand the role of the kidneys in the human body—how it functions, and how it can malfunction. Humans have two kidneys as part of their renal system (though in truth, they can function with only one), a system which also includes the ureters, bladder, and urethra—all of which are extremely important when talking about kidney stones and overall health. The ureters connect the kidneys to the bladder, while the urethra sits at the bottom part of the bladder and allows urine to exit the body.

The kidneys are responsible for filtering waste products out of the body. It does this through the use of hundreds of thousands of tiny filtering units called nephrons, which work through use of a special process to clean your blood of any undesirable substances while retaining those beneficial and necessary elements. **Kidney stones** are an abnormality that can be caused by an atypical response to unwanted substances in the body. These are hard mineral deposits that form inside your kidneys and obstruct the natural flow of blood through the renal system. The term used for the formation of a kidney stone is **nephrolithiasis**.

Having a kidney stone (also called calculus/calculi) is an experience you won't soon forget. They are extremely unpleasant and can drive people right to the floor from the pain. For this reason alone, it is important that you visit a urologist—a kidney/urinary specialist— if you think you could have a kidney stone.

Who is susceptible to kidney stones?

Anyone—of any race, color, or gender—can have kidney stones, but those born biologically male are more likely to experience them than those born female. In addition, people with high blood pressure, diabetes, and/or obesity are more likely to have kidney stones. However, it is still possible to have a kidney stone without any of these risk factors. Thankfully, certain health and lifestyle choices can greatly reduce your risk of developing a kidney stone.[2]

Are kidney stones genetic?

While genetics do play a significant role in the illnesses that we experience over our lifetime, and it would seem that kidney stones have a genetic component, it is currently unknown if they are passed down from generation (parents to children) or skip a generation (from grandparents to grandchildren skipping children).

What are kidney stones?

To discuss these in greater detail, a kidney stone is a salt and mineral deposit found in the urine and is made up of a wealth of different types of chemicals drawn from the foods we eat.

It is a small (though it seems rather large when it's moving around and you're trying to pass it!) object that forms starting in the kidney, where it then has to make its way out of the body by traveling out of the kidney, down the ureter, through the bladder, and out the urethra—that is, if they are able to be passed on their own at all.

How big are kidney stones?

Kidney stones are usually measured in millimeters (mm) and vary in size, and can range from smaller than 5mm to almost 10mm. A stone bigger than 5mm is more difficult to pass than 2mm, but both could require some type of intervention depending on where the stone is located, the type of stone, the patient's medical history, etc. Smaller stones *may* be able to be passed on their own; however, patients may not want to wait the potentially long span of time required, depending on how much pain they are in and other symptoms they are experiencing. This is completely understandable: imagine having something the size of a quarter stuck somewhere in your body, moving around every time you move or urinate. Making matters worse, kidney stones (no matter the size) can get stuck anywhere in the urinary tract, leading to difficulties passing urine and extreme pain.

So now that we have a better understanding of what a kidney stone is, how and where it forms, and why we certainly don't want to have one ourselves if we can at all avoid it, let's take a closer look at the conditions under which the various types of kidney stones form, to help pinpoint the risk factors we might be facing.

3

Symptoms and Types of Kidney Stones

TYPICALLY, A person's first hint that they are suffering from kidney stones will be a sharp, piercing pain in your side that doesn't go away with time. But not all kidney stones are large enough to cause this kind of noticeable pain; some are so small that they'll pass through your entire urinary system without you being any the wiser.

However, in the event that you aren't so lucky, let's go over the common (and uncommon) symptoms of kidney stones, as well as outline the various types of stones and their differences.

COMMON SYMPTOMS OF KIDNEY STONES

In addition to their debilitating and often extremely painful nature, additional symptoms that could signal a possible kidney stone include:

- Painful urination or a burning sensation while urinating

- Urine discoloration (may be cloudy)

- Changes in smell of urine

- Back/side/flank pain (intensity can come and go, unable to find comfortable position)

- Frequent urination

- Inability to pass urine

- Nausea/vomiting

- Blood in urine (hematuria)

- Frequent urinary tract infections

- Fever

- Chills

TYPES OF KIDNEY STONES

Once you and your doctor have established whether or not your symptoms are due to kidney stones or kidney stone complications, you'll next need to determine which type of stone you're afflicted with. There are several types of kidney stones, primarily differentiated by their root causes and specifics about their mineral make-up. In general, kidney stones form when substances in the urine are unable to be dissolved, but just *what* substances are involved will vary depending on the type of stone.

Calcium Oxalate Kidney Stones

Calcium oxalate kidney stones are the most common type of kidney stones and can be caused by not drinking enough water, having inadequate amounts of calcium or citrate in the body, and/or by consuming too many foods high in oxalates which in turn causes stone formation.

Foods high in oxalates include, but are not limited to:

- Beans and other legumes

- Beer

- Certain types of chocolate

- Coffee

- Potato chips and French fries

- Berries and cranberries

- Dark green vegetables, such as spinach

With this type of kidney stone, calcium binds to oxalate found in the urine to create the small, pain-inducing deposits.

Calcium Phosphate Kidney Stones

Calcium phosphate kidney stones are less common, as these occur only when your urinary system isn't functioning properly. According to the Mayo Clinic, some calcium phosphate kidney stones form due to the parathyroid glands being overactive. These glands are located on each of the four corners of the thyroid gland. When too much is secreted, it can lead to hyperthyroidism, causing an abundance of calcium in the body. Talk to your doctor about different treatment options for calcium phosphate stones.

Uric Acid Kidney Stones

Uric acid kidney stones are more likely to occur in men and are often associated with people who suffer from gout and/ or have a diet high in animal protein. Gout occurs when uric acid builds up in the joints causing pain, redness, inflammation, and tenderness. In certain cases, particularly when the afore-mentioned conditions are present, this uric acid build-up can carry over into the urinary system, resulting in the hard, painful abnormalities we call kidney stones.

Other people who are more susceptible to this type of stone include people who have received chemotherapy and who have a family history of uric acid kidney stones, meaning genetics may well play a factor in this type of stone.

Struvite Kidney Stones

Struvite kidney stones are more likely to be found in women, and originate from previous urinary tract infections. Struvite stones can grow to much larger size than other types of stones, which can cause further urinary problems if not treated quickly. Larger stones may not be able to be passed on their own and may require some form of intervention. Struvite kidney stones contain magnesium, ammonium, and phosphate, and form from having a bacterial infection. Ammonia raises the pH of urine, making it more alkaline (base). This can lead to kidney stones due to substances being unable to dissolve in alkaline urine.

Cystine Kidney Stones

Cystine kidney stones are the rarest type of kidney stones, and are caused by a specific illness called **cystinuria**. This disorder causes too much cystine in the urine, which leads to kidney stones. While rare, this is a lifelong condition and tends to run in families. As such, kidney stones caused by this disorder are typically recurring, and will need to be addressed regularly to ensure a pain-free quality of life.

While kidney stone pain is usually in the back, that isn't always the case. The location of your pain will depend on where the kidney stone is located and how your body responds to the pain. This, in turn, can lead to difficulties in diagnosis. For example, if the kidney stone is in the bladder, it could be mistaken as interstitial cystitis. It is possible to have pain in the abdomen, which could bring on gynecological diagnoses instead of properly diagnosing a kidney stone. It's important that proper testing is done to ensure the correct illness or ailment is diagnosed.

Samantha's Experience

According to my parents and sister, during the lithotripsy, my urologist removed pieces of the kidney stone they'd extracted and sent it off for testing to find out what type of stone I'd had. Unfortunately, when I went to my follow-up appointment two weeks later, the doctor told me that this in fact had *not* been done. I was understandably upset by this: knowing what type of stone I'd had would have been very helpful in making necessary diet changes to avoid having to go through this a second time. Still, I decided not to push the issue at the time because frankly, I was angry, frustrated, and in pain. I'm only human; I have my breaking point, too.

As it turned out, though, I probably should have pressed him on this. The *day* after the appointment, I received a bill in the mail from pathology, charging me for the expense of testing my kidney stone. I went straight to my urologist's office and demanded to know why I was told my stone wasn't tested, only to receive a bill telling me otherwise. The urologist apologized and told me that he'd forgotten—he *had* sent my stone off for testing, and then gave me a printout of the information he'd received and what foods I should be avoiding in the future. It absolutely floors me to know that a health professional can go into a patient's room without even looking at their charts beforehand. I understand that doctors have a lot of patients and these things can happen, but even with all of that, I don't feel like it excuses letting anyone's healthcare fall through the cracks. It just goes to show once again the paramount importance of persisting as your own healthcare advocate in every area of your treatment.

The urologist found that my stone had a diameter of five millimeters and was made of calcium oxalate. It showed little sign of infection, but if left untreated it could have caused serious problems. After all, kidney stones are foreign objects that don't belong in the body and the body is fighting to get it out any way it can. To that point, it had widened by two millimeters in just four weeks, and was causing horrible pain as well as urinary tract infections. At that point, my stone was the size of about the thickness of three quarters.

UNCOMMON SYMPTOMS

Depending on the type of kidney stone, its cause, and how long it has been left untreated, patients may experience complications including, but not limited to, sepsis, organ injury, needing blood transfusions, and neurogenic bladder. Sepsis occurs when chemicals are released in the body causing an inflammation response to spread throughout the system, harming instead of healing. Sepsis can be deadly and can be caused by any type of infection left untreated. Organs that are close to your kidney stone can be injured during surgery. Blood transfusions may be needed if there is a lot of bleeding that is hard to control. Neurogenic bladder occurs when nerves of the urinary system aren't working properly. It's important to see your doctor as soon as possible when you have a health concern, especially an infection. (You can learn more from NYU Lagone Health[3] and the National Kidney Foundation.)[4]

4

Testing and Treatment Options

WITH ALL the different types of kidney stones—and the wide range of other conditions that can present with side or flank pain—it's best to be sure that what you're suffering from *is* a kidney stone. Getting a correct diagnosis as soon as possible is key to a swift recovery from any illness, and kidney stones are no exception.

So, how do we determine whether a person has a kidney stone?

TESTING PROCEDURES FOR KIDNEY STONES

Testing is the first step in finding out what's going on if you're experiencing symptoms of a kidney infection or kidney stones. It's crucial you and your doctor first get a picture of what's going on in your body, especially before considering any type of surgery.

Urine Tests

The easiest and least invasive way to find out if you have a kidney infection is to have your doctor do a **urine test**. This test can be done in the doctor's office and you'll usually get the results during that same appointment. There are also over-the-counter strips that can be purchased to test your urine on your own at home. If the test comes back positive, call your doctor and ask them if they can fit you in for further testing and treatment.

Imaging Scans

Other procedures for detecting kidney stones are more invasive than urine testing is. Some procedures for detecting kidney stones include computed tomography (CT) scans, ultrasounds, and magnetic resonance imaging (MRI).

CT scans use x-rays to render 3-dimensional images of your urinary system including the kidneys, ureters, and bladder. This has the unfortunate side effect of exposing patients to high levels of radiation and it's important to know this when making your decision. CT scans also may involve drinking a contrast dye to help make sure the results of the test are more accurate and easy to read, though this will depend on exactly what your doctor is looking for.

Ultrasounds use sound waves to make an image of whatever organs are being scanned. The kidneys and bladder are scanned by an ultrasound technician just by putting the scanner over the organ, externally. There's no need for any contrast dye or IV, and there is no risk of radiation.

MRIs are scans that measure the response of atomic nuclei of body tissue to radio waves in a strong magnetic field. This creates an image of the internal organs that are scanned. MRIs usually take longer than CT scans but don't give off as much radiation. However, an MRI may involve needing an IV for contrast dye depending on what your doctor suspects is going on.

No matter what procedure is used, your doctor will need to use their discretion as to which test they think is the best fit for your case. However, just remember that you still have the final say as to whether or not you have a scan done, so be sure to do your research and weigh all your options.

TREATMENT OPTIONS

While it would be convenient to have some simple, over-the-counter pill to take that could dissolve the kidney stone and help it painlessly dissipate in the body, no such miracle drug exists. When faced with a kidney stone, there are realistically only two options: let nature take its course (i.e., let the stone pass naturally through your urine) or, if that isn't feasible, opt for a surgical procedure. As there really isn't much to be said about doing nothing and hoping for the best, we'll be focusing our attention on the surgical options.

There are several different types of surgeries for kidney stones and kidneys in general. Kidney stones usually don't cause damage, but the faster they are able to exit the body, the better. If left untreated over time, they can cause scarring, leading to other significant issues. For this reason, surgery may be required if the kidney stone isn't moving or else is stuck in place. That said, any type of surgery is still considered a trauma to the body. It's important that we remember this when making health care decisions and healing.

Nephrectomy

A **nephrectomy** is the removal of one or both kidneys. This usually isn't necessary for someone who is only presenting for the first time with a kidney stone, but may be considered in an extreme case, or if there is an extensive history of kidney stones.

Lithotripsy

Lithotripsy is a form of surgery performed by a urologist that uses sound waves to break up a kidney stone. According to the National Kidney Foundation, "Shock wave lithotripsy is the most common treatment of kidney stones in the United States."[5] During this procedure, shock waves are sent from outside of the body to the kidney stone so that it will fragment, be crushed, or bust into smaller pieces.

This procedure is usually done as outpatient, meaning the patient will not have to stay the night. This will, however, depend on how the patient responds, and can vary depending on guidelines for a patient's insurance plan. The patient will be put under general anesthesia, the lithotripsy will be performed, and a ureteral stent will most likely be inserted during the procedure. This is a thin tube placed in your ureter, with one end inside your kidney and the other end in your bladder. This serves to bridge these parts of the urinary system to help drain urine from your kidney and has the added benefit of helping remove any leftover fragments from the stone pass without blockages or any other problems.

Some types of stones will respond better than others to lithotripsy, so it's important that your doctor evaluates you and your kidney stone before deciding on treatment. You will not have any incisions having a lithotripsy performed. If you had a ureteral stent inserted during the procedure, the performing physician will remove the stent anywhere from three days to three months after insertion depending on the reason the stent was placed. Some stents even have a string on the end to make it easier to remove. The Urology Care Foundation defines a stent as "a soft, hollow, plastic tube placed in the ureter, with the top portion of the stent having a small curl that sits in the kidney and the opposite end curls in the bladder. [6]

Your doctor should talk to you about the risks involved in this procedure. You can also ask how many lithotripsy procedures they've done in the past and how often they see these risks present in their cases. Potential risks of lithotripsy include infection rate, kidney stones blocking urine from exiting the body, and bleeding risks. Depending on how serious these complications are, more measures and/or interventions may be necessary.

Nephrolithotomy

A **nephrolithotomy** is a surgery in which a surgeon makes incisions on the patient's back to get a better look and feel for the state of the kidney. A scope is inserted into the incision to remove any kidney stones that are unable to pass on their own and which do not stand to benefit from a lithotripsy. This surgery can be helpful for patients who have diverticulum on their kidneys where the kidney stones are trapped and unable to exit the body on their own.

Potential complications of a nephrolithotomy include blood in the urine, as well as kidney pain and back pain related to the surgery; the latter of which should decrease within a couple of days. This is a less common surgery than lithotripsy and it's important that your doctor feels comfortable in performing the nephrolithotomy and is certain that it's best for your health.

Nephrostomy

A **nephrostomy** is a procedure wherein a surgeon makes an opening between the skin and the kidney, after which a nephrostomy tube is placed from the back into the kidney to help urine pass. This can be used for kidney stones, depending on their location, and will usually be placed by a radiologist, who will use imaging techniques to determine where to place the tube.

Potential risks from this surgery include a high fever, infection, pain in your lower back, blood in your urine, and pulmonary complications such as fluid around the lungs. If any of these occur, other interventions may be necessary. If fluid collects and builds up around the lungs, a chest tube may also need to be inserted to drain the fluid. Be sure to cover all the risks associated before deciding to have this or any type of surgery. In particular, ask your doctor if they're equipped to handle these complications or if there's someone they would be able to quickly refer you to for help.

Diverticulum Interventions

Diverticula are unwanted outpouchings found on the kidney that affect the upper collecting system. They can wreak havoc on the kidneys and your overall health and may require some type of intervention. There are several treatment options available to practitioners for the treatment of diverticula, such as glue or electrical fulguration, which allow them to close the outpouchings and minimize stone formation and infection. **Electrical fulguration** involves making an incision at the neck of the diverticulum using low-current electrocautery. Once this is done, a nephrostomy tube will be required for a couple of days. A scan called a nephrostogram will also be performed to determine if there are any stone fragments left; if everything is clear, the nephrostomy tube can be removed. This type of scan is conducted by the radiology department and also shows how the kidneys are functioning.[7]

Be sure to talk to your doctors about any risks that are involved with any surgeries or procedures they recommend. It's important that you weigh the risks against the benefits of any procedure before giving your consent. Don't let a doctor pressure you into taking medications or having surgeries done, or assigning you any other form of treatment you don't feel comfortable with. Some surgery recoveries are harder than others and it's important to remember that everyone's experience is different. However, it's important that we feel supported no matter what our experience.

Samantha's Experience
I'd had a CT scan and an ultrasound the first time I went to the emergency room complaining of pain from my kidney stone and infection. Thankfully, I

didn't have to drink any contrast fluid for these, nor did I need to have any MRIs related to my kidneys or bladder during this time. I knew the radiation risk of having any number of CT scans done, but I felt like it was necessary given what I was going through to find the right answer, quickly.

These tests were sufficient to determine that the source of my pain was a kidney stone, but unfortunately the only way to identify which *type* of kidney stone is involved is by testing a piece of the stone, which in my case could only be obtained from surgery. Couple this with my horrible pain, urinary symptoms, and my being unable to pass the stone on my own, it became clear that I needed to have surgery. I underwent lithotripsy about four weeks after my first emergency room visit, which was an extremely long month to be in constant pain. I also took some time off work because I knew from previous experiences my sister had that I would still be in some pain following the lithotripsy.

The doctors stuck me for an IV to give me fluids and medications, and while I couldn't eat or drink anything after midnight prior to the procedure, I thankfully didn't need to do a bowel prep. My parents and sister went with me and stayed in the waiting room to talk to my doctor after he finished the procedure, which was completed without complication. My doctor was able to go in and break up my kidney stone, remove the fragments, and insert a stent to make sure I was still able to urinate properly. Even better, I didn't have any problems with my bladder "waking up" after surgery and was able to urinate on my own without a catheter. (In the past, there were several times I had to be catheterized because my bladder wouldn't function or empty on its own after sedation, even though I could feel that I needed to urinate.) I did wake up with some pain, not in my back or kidney, but in my urethra, even though the stent went from my right kidney to my bladder by way of my ureter.

While I've personally never had any horrible reactions or problems waking up when under anesthesia, there have been times when I was put to sleep and was prescribed a scopolamine patch to go behind my ear. This is intended to help with the nausea when you wake up, and if this is something you think would be helpful for you, ask your anesthesiologist about whether this is something they can do. (Note that scopolamine side effects can include dry mouth, sleepiness, and agitation, so be sure to do your own research to make sure this is the best option for you and your surgery needs.)

I had my stent removed two weeks after having lithotripsy. I remember lying in my bed for many hours if not most of the day in so much pain, setting my alarm to take my medication right on time because I was afraid that if I didn't take it like clockwork my pain would intensify to the point of becoming uncontrollable. In fact, the stent removal was the worst part of having lithotripsy surgery for me. I was prescribed Pyridium (three times daily) to help with kidney spasms, Keflex as an antibiotic (four times daily), and Norco (four times daily) for pain. I finished the Norco prescription in five days and the antibiotic in a week, but after I ran out I was still in a lot of pain so I called my doctor to see if I could get more. Unfortunately, they wouldn't prescribe me anymore and couldn't see me sooner to remove my stent. I also couldn't work with the amount of pain I was experiencing, which was very frustrating and discouraging. I even used a heating pad for my abdomen to try and help with some of the discomfort I was experiencing.

I was still in pain a week after having my stent removed, but at least I was able to go back to work. At least, I was for the three hours I was scheduled for—I had to cancel my next shift two days later because of how much pain I was in.

About three weeks after my kidney stone procedure and one week after my stent was removed, it was back to the emergency room for me. My vitals were normal, my scans were clear, and my blood work came back normal, but a urine test showed I had a urinary tract infection. Either the antibiotics I was prescribed after the lithotripsy didn't get rid of it, or the infection had come back. I called to schedule an appointment with my doctor, but they didn't call me back until after I was at the emergency room and said they would have called me in an antibiotic without being seen. I had no idea if they were going to call me back and by this time I was very frustrated with my experiences with this doctor office. At the emergency room, I was immediately called back because they weren't busy.

A month later, I was still experiencing pain. I decided to make an appointment with another urologist, one further away, whom my sister had seen for extensive kidney surgeries and recommended. My current urologist kept insisting that the pain and symptoms I was experiencing were just from surgery, but by this time, my lithotripsy was two months ago; it just didn't make sense to me that my pain would still be from the procedure.

I went in for my appointment and had my urine tested. He asked me about my symptoms: I was still experiencing back pain on my right side in the same area, nausea, frequent urination, and sometimes burning feelings with urination. He prescribed me Bactrim, which is in a class of antibiotics I hadn't tried yet, and agreed with me that I shouldn't still be experiencing these symptoms after surgery. I felt relieved to have my symptoms and experiences validated by someone who could help me. I took the prescription for two weeks and it cleared up my urinary tract infection.

Yet a few days after seeing my new urologist, I needed to go to the emergency room for a fourth time—the fourth visit in four months—because I was once again in extreme pain. I suspected it was a kidney stone because I was experiencing the same pain I'd had before my surgery. When the doctor finally came in and talked things over with me, he recommended we not have a CT scan performed and suggested that we have blood work done and an ultrasound of my kidneys had instead, as this would be safer. The bloodwork showed my liver enzymes were elevated again, with an AST of 592, an ALT of 466, and alkaline phosphatase at 144. I still wasn't sure if this had to do with my kidney stone, but I hadn't been taking any medications other than antibiotics so I had no idea what was going on.

The emergency room doctor suggested that I have an ultrasound of my liver done along with my kidneys. This confirmed that I *didn't* have additional kidney stones, but that still left me needing to figure out what was going on with my liver. Being part of the chronic illness community, I knew of conditions that could be causing my liver issues. Meanwhile, I was feeling very upset because I felt like I was still having to wait for answers while being scared of what they could be. I began to wonder if my liver issues had been causing my symptoms all along, and the first emergency room visit had just happened to find a kidney stone, as the pain never really went away in my back or side. This is why it is so difficult to deal with chronic health conditions. Chronic pain can change a person. It's important that we have people in our lives we can talk to about our feelings; for example, having a therapist can be helpful. It's crucial that we find things that can help decrease our stress and help us relax like warm baths and reading. Our mental health is just as important as our physical health.

As of the middle of 2020, I've not had any additional complications that would suggest further kidney stones, so hopefully this marks the end of my journey with this condition. I'm very thankful that I didn't require any other interventions and hope that I don't require any in the future.

NON-SURGICAL TREATMENT OPTIONS

While there is no magic pill for kidney stones, aside from surgery there are several potential treatments that may be helpful for passing your kidney stone, depending on its size, location, and other factors. Leave no stone unturned when researching, if you'll pardon the pun.

Antibiotics

Antibiotics are a class of medication which kill bacteria and are used to treat infections. Different families of antibiotics are used for different strains of bacteria, though they've been receiving scrutiny in recent years because of how they negatively interfere with our internal microbiome. It's important when taking an antibiotic to finish the entire prescription as it's prescribed by your doctor. Stopping early can allow the bacteria to resurge within you.

> *Samantha's Experience*
>
> During the span of time I was seeking treatment for my kidney stone, I was on several antibiotics to help eradicate my kidney infection/urinary tract infection, including Cipro, Keflex, and Bactrim. I noticed the largest relief with Bactrim; Cipro and Keflex both helped with my symptoms somewhat, but the infection itself never went away. I was prescribed these separately and took them 2–4 times daily for up to two weeks. I chose to take these antibiotics because my infections weren't going to go away on their own, unfortunately.

There are several types of antibiotics, some of which can be found in the table below. Please note that the Potential Side

Effects column is by no means an extensive or complete list. Be sure to do your own research to determine side effects and properly weigh the risks against the benefits. Just because a medication can have a certain side effect, doesn't mean you will suffer with it. However, it does mean that it's a possibility and you have a right to know that. It's important that you know all the facts before agreeing to any form of treatment.

Class of Antibiotic	Medications	Use	Potential Side Effects
Penicillin	Penicillin Amoxicillin	Wide variety of infections, including kidney infections	Diarrhea, allergic reaction, skin rash, itching, peeling
Tetracyclines	Tetracycline Doxycycline	Skin infections Acne	Nausea, vomiting, diarrhea, loss of appetite
Cephalosporins	Keflex Cefdinir	Wide variety of infections including kidney infections	Nausea, vomiting, stomach discomfort, thrush, rash
Quinolones (Fluoroquinolones)	Ciprofloxacin	Urinary tract infections	Nausea, vomiting, dizziness, insomnia (trouble with sleep)
Lincomycin	Lincomycin	A narrow spectrum antibiotic used for patients who can't take Penicillin antibiotics	Diarrhea, stomach pain, nausea, vomiting, vaginal itching

Class of Antibiotic	Medications	Use	Potential Side Effects
Macro-lides	Azithromy-cin Clari-thromycin	Wide variety of infections in-cluding kidney infections	Nausea, vom-iting, diarrhea, allergic reac-tion, buzzing in ears (tinnitus)
Sulfon-amides	Bactrim Septra Sulfame-thoxaz-ole-tri-methoprim derivatives	Wide variety of infections in-cluding kidney infections	Skin rash, dizzi-ness, headache, diarrhea Some people are allergic to this class of antibiotics, possibly be-cause they are synthetic and a mixture of chemicals.
Glyco-peptides	Vancomycin (IV only)	Staph (MRSA) infections	Nausea, diar-rhea, vomit-ing, headache, dizziness, foamy urine
Amino-glycosides	Gentamycin	Broad spectrum used if other antibiotics don't eradicate kid-ney infection	Loss of hear-ing, ringing or buzzing in ears, skin rash, increased thirst

Class of Antibiotic	Medications	Use	Potential Side Effects
Carbap-enems	Imipenem Meropenem	High risk infections/used when other antibiotics don't work on killing bacteria (also known as multidrug-resistant)	Nausea, vomiting, diarrhea, rash, headache
Nitrofu-rans	Macrobid	Kidney infections Kidney stones	Diarrhea, sudden chest pain, fever, chills, body aches, numbness

Probiotics

According to the National Center for Complementary and Integrative Health, **probiotics** are live microorganisms that are intended to have health benefits when consumed or applied to the body.[8] These benefits can include helping your body maintain a healthy community of microorganisms or helping your body's community of microorganisms return to a healthy condition after being disturbed, as well as positively influence your body's immunity response.[8] In other words, you can take probiotics to help replenish your store of bacteria that are beneficial to the body.

Samantha's Experience

As for probiotics, I've tried many different types since being diagnosed with irritable bowel syndrome to try to help relieve my stomach issues. I tried many that were available over-the-counter, but I never really noticed a difference. It wasn't until 2018 that I came across a probiotic from Shaklee that a friend recommended, and that's helped me a lot. However, during the time of my kidney stone and liver issues, I decided to stop everything else I was on and only take the antibiotics, as I didn't know what was and wasn't affecting my liver. Stopping the probiotic resulted in no noticeable changes to my symptoms, however, and even if it had, I could still have chosen to take the probiotic several hours apart from the antibiotic.

Probiotics shouldn't be taken at the same time as antibiotics; rather, a probiotic should always be taken several hours before or after an antibiotic. Even though probiotics are available over-the-counter and don't require a prescription, it's still important to let your doctors know that you are taking one so they are aware and can make a note of it.

It's worth mentioning that the U.S. Food and Drug Administration (FDA) doesn't regulate supplements like probiotics, unlike prescription medications, which do need to be approved by the FDA. However, it's also worth noting that this has not stopped prescriptions being written for conditions based on little scientific information, often with potentially horrible side effects.

Alternate Medications

Perhaps you've decided that antibiotics aren't for you. After all, there have been studies that have suggested that oral antibiotics can actually *increase* the risk of kidney stones. So where does this leave you for treating a kidney stone or infection? In addition to diet changes and over-the-counter products, consider some of the following. In the table below, you will find some medications that may be helpful in treating kidney infections and kidney stones. Again, the Potential Side Effects column is not an extensive list, and just because a medication *can* have a certain side effect doesn't mean you *will* suffer from it. However, it does mean that it's a possibility and it's important that you have all the facts before agreeing to any form of treatment.

Name of Medication	Use	Potential Side Effects
Flomax (Generic: Tamsulosin)	A prescription that can be used to treat kidney stones as well as enlarged prostate because it increases urinary frequency. This may be prescribed to help someone pass a kidney stone because the medication relaxes the bladder (and prostate in men).	Nausea, diarrhea, dizziness, drowsiness, weakness, back pain

Name of Medication	Use	Potential Side Effects
AZO/Pyridium	Can be used to help relieve urinary pain. AZO can be purchased over-the-counter while Pyridium requires a prescription from a doctor. This may be prescribed while trying to pass a kidney stone on your own or after lithotripsy to help with the stent pain and urinary system spasms.	Swelling, weight gain, confusion, loss of appetite These medications may turn the urine orange or a different color from clear/yellow. It's important to know this ahead of time before taking it so it doesn't cause concern.
Toradol (Ketorolac tromethamine) Aleve (Naproxen) Tylenol (Acetaminophen) Motrin (Ibuprofen) NSAIDs	NSAIDs can help with pain caused by kidney stones.	Toradol: Headache, heartburn, nausea, vomiting, diarrhea Aleve: indigestion, heartburn, stomach pain, headache, dizziness, drowsiness Tylenol: liver issues, skin reactions Ibuprofen: stomach issues, headache, dizziness, rash, itching NSAIDs: stomach ulcers, diarrhea, nausea, bloating, constipation

Name of Medication	Use	Potential Side Effects
Methylene Blue	Used for patients that have a history of kidney stone formation to try to help prevent more stones from forming	Bladder irritation, dizziness, headache, sweating, nausea, vomiting
Pain medications (Norco, etc.)	Acute (short term) pain relief	Dizziness, drowsiness, itching, nausea, vomiting

Be sure to ask your doctor about any drug side effects and interactions and do your own research to make sure you choose the best treatment option for yourself.

Samantha's Experience

In addition to antibiotics, I tried and was prescribed a number of both prescription and over-the-counter medications in hopes of relieving my symptoms.

AZO is an over-the-counter supplement that I started taking when I first found out I had a kidney stone because it's supposed to help with urinary symptoms. I decided to take AZO because I was having a lot of urinary pain and burning, to the point that I dreaded going to the bathroom. It turned my urine orange, which I knew to expect, and it also helped with some of the burning I was experiencing when urinating. I usually took it every eight hours as needed. Be sure to follow the directions on the box of AZO you purchase, as they make different strengths which carry different instructions.

The urologist who performed my lithotripsy prescribed **Pyridium** for me to take alongside **Norco** for the pain of both the procedure and the stent. As a stent is essentially a foreign object, it's understandable and the body really doesn't want it there, and the body's response to this unwelcome guest is to cause inflammation and pain. Pyridium turned my urine orange, as expected, and it did help with the burning feeling I had when urinating. I took this medication three times every day for almost two weeks, until I ran out. I actually ran out of both Pyridium and Norco before I had my stent removed, which was extremely painful to deal with. I decided to take Pyridium because it was similar to AZO and it seemed to help with the burning and spasm pain that I was experiencing.

I was prescribed **Flomax** the second time I went to the emergency room, as it was expected that Flomax would help me urinate more, which could in theory help me pass the kidney stone. I *did* urinate more frequently, but I still wasn't able to pass my kidney stone on my own. I decided to take Flomax because at this time, I needed help with urinating and I seemed to be unable to completely empty my bladder on my own. I also knew that this could be dangerous if nothing was done.

During most of my visits to the emergency room, I received **Toradol** injected into my IV for pain and inflammation, and each time I received it, it helped decrease my pain significantly. Before I went to the emergency room the first time, I'd taken Percocet for the pain that I had from a previous surgery, but it didn't touch the pain I was experiencing. But while there *is* a tablet form of Toradol, hospitals rarely give it to patients to take home, as Toradol isn't really a long-term solution, but more of a band-aid. As a side note, any time that I take a pain medicine that is a controlled substance like Norco or Percocet, I have to take Benadryl with it to combat the itching that these pain medications can cause. There have been times when I would take the medication without Benadryl and I would feel like I needed to scratch my face off. Of course, taking Benadryl with Norco or Percocet causes even more drowsiness so talk to your doctor before adding Benadryl to your regimen. Even without Benadryl, the drowsiness caused by these medications is significant; on days when I had to work, I would take Aleve instead of Norco to help with the pain and inflammation because I didn't feel like I should drive while taking Norco. Be sure to read all warnings that come with any medication you take and make these decisions for yourself. Be sure to talk to your doctor if you experience itching or other side effects.

On the topic of side effects, nausea and bowel issues are among the most common symptoms of painkillers, but I've suffered with those issues for a long time so it's hard for me to know if any of the medications caused or increased these symptoms for me. Likewise, I've never really had bad headaches and didn't have any while taking any of these medications, but that is my own personal experience. I also couldn't know beforehand if any of these medications would cause side effects in my body, but I still weighed out my risks versus having relief, taking into account available research, and in the end chose to take the medications I did. This process will be different for each individual and health decisions shouldn't be made quickly (unless necessary) or taken lightly.

Finally, a general word of caution: pain medicine carries its own risks. Things like Tylenol can damage your liver, while other medications can be addictive, and I don't just mean chemically. Being in that much pain—pain that's truly off the charts—can drive you to desperation. Living with chronic illnesses, I know that I'm never going to be completely pain-free, which means I *do* need some type of pain relief to function. But while drugs like Norco can be addictive—I'm sure that's why my first urologist wouldn't write me another prescription—Toradol and Aleve don't fall into this category. Aleve, Naproxen, Motrin, and other medications like them are available in over-the-counter and prescription strength, and due to their different chemical composition, they have less potential to become addictive.

In the next chapter, we'll take a look at some of the risk factors associated with developing kidney stones or having chronic kidney concerns, as well as what steps you can take to help mitigate these risks.

5

Genetics

O **UR GENETICS** play a huge part in our overall health. They determine our chances of developing certain types of disorders as well as affect how our bodies reacts to specific illness, including the development of kidney stones. Genetics also play a role in who develops certain types of kidney stones, as certain varieties of kidney stones are directly linked to either one's genetic makeup, or their risk of developing specific inherited illnesses. It's important to ask your family questions about their health so you can get an idea of what they've been through and some things you should look out for.

Medical science is still undecided on the exact role and impact of genetics in the development of kidney stones, with some medical professionals believing kidney stones go right down the line of a family (grandparent to parent to child) while others believe it skips a generation (grandparent to grandchild). In other words, while we *do* know that they run in families, your parents or other relatives having a certain illness doesn't automatically mean you have or will have that illness. What it *does* mean is that you are at an increased risk of certain illnesses.

Thankfully, the risks of some illnesses with genetic components, kidney stones included, can be decreased by diet changes. More information on the steps you can take to minimize your risk of developing kidney stones can be found in the following chapter.

Some other health conditions which can make people more prone to developing kidney stones include hypercalciuria (too much calcium in the urine), hypocitraturia (not enough citrate in the urine), primary hyperoxaluria (the result of a gene mutation that causes a defect in liver enzyme and excretion of too much oxalate), and cystinuria.

Samantha's Experience

I'm not the only person in my family to have developed kidney stones: my sister has had many kidney stones, involving a host of procedures, surgical interventions, and complications, and my brother has experienced many kidney stones that he's been able to pass on his own. My extended family suffers from kidney stones, too, both on my mother's and father's sides. However, neither of my parents has experienced kidney stones (to our knowledge) and, as far as we know, my grandparents, aunts, and uncles haven't, either.

In other words, it seems as though kidney stones have skipped a generation in my family. But this may not be the case for everyone; as well, more research is needed in this area to really nail down how big a part our genetics play. I recommend you and your families keep each other informed on any past or present health concerns. I know some issues can be embarrassing (like irritable bowel syndrome), but it can be helpful to talk about them with family members so that they can get a glimpse into what you're going through, as well as keep an eye out for themselves if it's something that runs in families.

6

Lifestyle Changes

M AKING HEALTHY lifestyle choices like keeping active and prioritizing a nutritious balanced diet can help prevent—and at times, even resolve—kidney stones. However, it is important to remember that making sudden or drastic lifestyle changes can do more harm than good, especially if you do so without understanding how those changes will interact with your specific illness. The following are some proven options that you can consider when trying to live a life free of kidney stone-related pain.

STAYING HYDRATED

Staying hydrated throughout the day is important for supporting all bodily functions. In the case of kidney stones, water can potentially flush the stone out (depending on its size and location). On the flip side, being dehydrated can actually *increase* your risk of developing a kidney stone, as well as decrease your odds of being able to pass it on your own. Harvard Health Publishing found that drinking two liters of fluid a day reduces the likelihood of stone recurrence by about half. Likewise, the American Urological Association guidelines for medical management of kidney stones recommends that patients who form kidney stones should aim to drink more than 2.5 liters of fluid per day.[9] Two liters comes out to be a little less than a gallon of water, and while drinking this much may have you running back and forth to the bathroom often, doing so will do a lot to help flush the toxins out of your system.

Remember: our body is about 60 percent water by weight, so it's important that we maintain our water intake. That's why when you go to the emergency room with symptoms of dehydration, they'll give you fluids such as saline through an IV to help. Symptoms of dehydration include not urinating enough, dark-colored urine, dizziness, and a fast heartbeat. People who are hydrated usually have light yellow or close to clear urine.

DIET CHANGES

Certain types of kidney stones are more likely to develop when your body contains an abundance (or overabundance) of certain minerals. For example, the most common type of kidney stone is composed of calcium oxalate, which is comprised of both calcium and oxalate, the latter of which is a natural substance present in many foods. In the case of kidney stones, the oxalate binds to calcium in the stomach and intestines during digestion and leaves the body in the form of stool. Any oxalate that is not bound to calcium travels as a waste product, moving from the blood to the kidneys where it leaves the body in the urine. If there is too much oxalate and too little liquid in the urine, calcium oxalate fragments are formed. As these fragments increase in number, they start to coalesce, clumping together to form the larger mass we know as a kidney stone.

Once you've determined what type of kidney stone you have, your doctor should be able to inform you as to whether there is any dietary component to consider. If so, they can provide you with a list of what foods you should avoid to prevent unwanted build-up in your kidneys.[10,11] Below is a table listing foods that contain low, medium and high oxalate content, which helps illustrate some of the dietary adjustments you might need to make if you develop calcium oxalate stones.

Type of Food	Low Oxalate	Medium Oxalate	High Oxalate
Beverages	Water Cider Coca-Cola Distilled alcohol Fruit juices Ginger ale Kukicha twig tea Lemonade Limeade (made with peel) Minute maid Orange soda Pepsi	Coffee Cranberry juice	Beer-lager draft, Tuborg, Pilsner Chocolate milk Juices with berries Ovaltine Tea, black, Indian Bigelow herbal teas (hot, brew time 4 minutes)
Fruits	Peeled apples Avocado Canned cranberries Coconut Cherries Green grapes Watermelon Bananas Cantaloupe Nectarines Raisins	Apples with skin Apricots Black currants Dried cranberries Grapefruit Oranges Peaches Pears Pineapple Plums Prunes	Blackberries Blueberries Dried Figs Gooseberries Kiwi Strawberries Tangerines Rhubarb Raspberries

Type of Food	Low Oxalate	Medium Oxalate	High Oxalate
Vegetables	Squash Alfalfa Cabbage Cauliflower Peas Red peppers Radishes Turnips, roots Zucchini	Asparagus Artichokes Brussels sprouts Broccoli Carrots Corn Peeled cucumbers Lettuce Lima beans Mushrooms	Celery Chives Dandelion Eggplant Kale Leeks Mustard greens Okra Parsley Parsnips Green peppers Vegetable soup Yams
Condiments	Ketchup Mustard Mayonnaise Others not listed in moderate or high oxalate columns	Fresh basil Malt, powder Pepper	Cinnamon Raw parsley Pepper Ginger Soy sauce
Dairy	Milk (skim, 2%, or whole) Buttermilk Yogurt with approved fruit	None	Chocolate milk
Fats and Oils	All oils	None	None

Type of Food	Low Oxalate	Medium Oxalate	High Oxalate
Grains, Breads, and Starches	Bread Cereals Egg or macaroni noodles White or wild rice	Cooked barley Corn bread Corn tortilla Cornmeal Cornstarch White or wheat flour Oatmeal Brown rice Sponge cake	Fig Newtons Fruit cake Graham crackers White corn grits Marmalade
Meats	Beef Lamb Pork Eggs Fish/shellfish Poultry	Beef kidney Liver	None
Meat Substitutes, Beans, Nuts, and Seeds	Eggs Lentils Water chestnuts	Canned garbanzo beans Lima beans Cooked split peas	Almonds Baked beans canned in tomato sauce Cashews Green beans Peanut butter Peanuts Pecans Sesame Seeds Sunflower Seeds Tofu Walnuts

It's important to note that just because a food is low in ox-alate, that doesn't mean you can or should eat as much of that food as you want. Keep serving sizes in mind when consuming any food. This list is not extensive, nor does it cover every type of kidney stone. These examples are spe-cifically given for the most common type of stone, calcium oxalate. You are encouraged to research information specific to your type of stone, making sure to draw on information from multiple vetted sources that you know and trust. For example, the urologist who performed my lithotripsy pro-vided me with a reference from North Austin Urology that I found quite helpful.[12] Do your own research; it's important to get information from multiple sources and compare sim-ilarities and differences. Use sources that are vetted and you know and trust. Specialist websites can be helpful, as well as medical colleges; if you see a website that is only for a certain treatment or medication, keep researching. It's also import-ant to note here that just because one treatment option did or didn't work for me, doesn't mean that the same treatment option will/won't work for you.

Be sure to talk to your doctor about how much protein and calcium you should be consuming to make sure you are getting an adequate amount of each and not too much. In addition to the above, the National Institute of Diabetes and Digestive Kidney Diseases (a subset of the National Institute of Health) provides many helpful dietary recommendations, which can be found both below and on their website:[13]

Calcium Phosphate

Reduce or avoid:

- Sodium and grease (salty fast foods)

- Animal protein (including beef, chicken, pork, eggs, fish, shellfish, milk, cheese, dairy products, etc.)

Prioritize:

- Legumes (beans, dried peas, lentils, peanuts)
- Soy foods (soy milk, soy nut butter, tofu)
- Nuts (almonds, almond butter, cashews, cashew butter, walnuts, pistachios)
- Sunflower seeds

Uric Acid

Reduce or avoid:

- Animal protein (including beef, chicken, pork, eggs, fish, shellfish, milk, cheese, dairy products, etc.)

Prioritize:

- Legumes (beans, dried peas, lentils, peanuts)
- Soy foods (soy milk, soy nut butter, tofu)
- Nuts (almonds, almond butter, cashews, cashew butter, walnuts, pistachios)
- Sunflower seeds

Samantha's Experience

Knowing what I know now, I'd never have expected a kidney stone—I drink more than enough water every day! When I was four or five years old, my grandma would babysit me and always had a big jug of water with her, and whenever I was thirsty, I would drink from it. As I got older, I never quite liked the way soda and milk made my stomach feel, so I just stuck with water.

Around the same time as my kidney stone, I was also making a point of eating more fruits and vegetables, which in most cases would be the healthy call to make, but it turns out that those vegetables (like asparagus and spinach) were contributing to my risk of developing stones. There are few things as frustrating as trying to do the right thing for your health, only to find out that it's been hurting you all along. It makes you feel like throwing your hands up in exasperation. As far as making dietary changes, I've incorporated the advice I got from the urologist to avoid any future stones, but even if I'd known the proper diet changes to make, it still wouldn't have helped me pass the stone I had; surgery would still have been my best option.

As far as how I've changed my diet now that I need to avoid high oxalate foods, it hasn't been easy. I've had to cut certain favorite foods out of my life and practice self-control. I have to continue reminding myself of the pain I experienced with my kidney stone and how important it is to my health that I stay away from high oxalate foods as much as possible. Some of the items that I have cut out of my personal diet include tea, peanuts, peanut butter, pecans, strawberries, blueberries, peaches, grits, green beans, celery, okra, and green peppers. I also tend to stay away from medium oxalate foods like asparagus and bacon. Safe foods that I continue to eat include green grapes, peeled apples, avocados, watermelon, white rice, beef, chicken, poultry, eggs, fish, peeled cucumbers, and lettuce.

Of course, it's not just a matter of choosing the right foods and avoiding the wrong ones. It is also important that I follow the proper serving sizes for these foods, as well as how they're prepared and seasoned. Thankfully, many condiments like ketchup are considered low oxalate and so I'm still able to enjoy those. But I have had to stop eating frozen foods like frozen pizzas, chicken alfredo, and lasagna because they tend to have higher amounts of sodium.

DIETARY SUPPLEMENTS

Low levels of vitamin D have been associated with kidney stone formation. This doesn't mean that every single person who has a vitamin D deficiency will have a kidney stone at some point in their life; this just means that having this deficiency increases one's risk of having kidney stones. There are different forms of vitamin D and different blood tests that can be done to check your levels. Talk to your doctor about testing and your levels before starting any supplementation. Vitamin D is important for so many things including bone health, heart health, and even kidney health.

There is also the option of seeing a nutritionist to help with diet changes. It can be helpful to have someone hold you accountable and to feel like you're not alone in making the necessary changes.

Samantha's Experience

When I first started getting my period, I was extremely tired and didn't feel like myself. At the time, I was a young teenager and it felt like I shouldn't be as tired as I was. After I turned 18, I was able to change doctors to one I felt would take my complaints more seriously, and my new doctor tested me to see what my vitamin D level was. The normal range is 50 and above; my initial level was in the 30s. I have been taking a vitamin D supplement pretty much ever since to try to keep my levels within the normal range. The last time I had my vitamin D level checked, it was back in the 50s—and that's from taking 5,000 IU daily.

It can be extremely difficult to give up your favorite foods, but just remember that your health is absolutely worth it. Without good health, it's impossible for us to function at our best. If we don't feel up to par, it affects every aspect of our lives. If you're really struggling with adjusting to a new diet, it can be helpful to focus on replacing foods rather than cutting them out. For example, if you're accustomed to drinking tea, rather than cutting it out and moving on, start drinking lemonade and cranberry juice instead. As an added plus, both are supposed to be good for getting rid of kidney stones and cleaning out the urinary tract!

In the next chapter, we'll go over the financial side of receiving treatment for kidney stones. Having a proper understanding and expectation of the costs involved can help you plan for the future, as well as provide you with one more good reason to do what it takes to avoid getting stones in the first place.

7

Medical Expenses and Costs

HEALTHCARE IS extremely expensive in the United States, even with insurance coverage. Chief among the issues involved is that insurance companies get to decide whether they will or won't cover the cost of a medication or procedure, all without any medical information about the policy holder or the illness being treated. Some insurance policies require prior authorization for certain treatments; others require that the patient try a different medication before they will cover what the doctor first prescribed. Needing prior authorization means the pharmacy needs to first contact the prescribing physician, who must then contact the insurance company to say the medication is medically necessary. Without this prior authorization, patients can pay cash for the treatment they need, but doing so will be very expensive. This forces the patient to wait days or even longer for medications and procedures that may be lifesaving.

Insurance companies never see the patient or know anything other than what comes up on a computer screen, yet they get to dictate what they will cover for a patient to receive treatment for a certain illness, regardless of whether it's acute or chronic. All the while, patients are paying monthly premiums on top of meeting deductibles just to have some type of medical coverage, only to then have certain treatments denied.

Long story short, it's critical that you understand, to the best of your ability, what your coverage will provide for and what you can financially afford. Failure to do so will quite literally cost you—and even with a relatively straightforward issue like kidney stones, there are quite a number of costs involved.

DOCTOR'S APPOINTMENTS

Urologists are doctors who specialize in all things urinary, which like any specialist means their fees may be more expensive than a family practitioner. Depending on your doctor's office and insurance, you may need to have your general practitioner or another doctor send the urologist a referral before you can schedule an appointment to be seen. Once you have the appointment, the urologist will talk to you and may want to order a series of tests (blood work, urine test, 24-hour urine test, MRI, CT scan, X-ray, and/or ultrasound) depending on what your situation is. Without insurance or financial assistance, one scan or X-ray can cost thousands of dollars depending on the facility.

LOST INCOME

It's important to note that anyone with a kidney stone will more than likely have to miss a number of days from work, school, or any other activities, whether they are trying to pass the kidney stone on their own or having surgery. This will affect their income and their ability to pay bills on time, as well as provide for their family. It's nearly impossible to perform all your normal daily functions while having a kidney stone, but it can be difficult to take time off of work when you don't have sick time or vacation time to use, just to make sure you have some type of income coming in. Know that you have to take care of yourself before you can take care of anyone else. Your health has to be a priority, even if other people in your life or at work don't understand or sympathize.

Samantha's Experience

Over the last 10 years, I have accumulated at least $100,000 worth of medical bills, some with medical insurance, some without. For my kidney stone in particular, I racked up about $28,000 worth of medical bills over the course of four hospital stays, five doctor's appointments, and related medications. This was with discounts for self-pay or cash-only patients. I don't mind telling you that having this much medical debt is extremely stressful and makes me not want to seek medical care even when I need it because I know other people are in this same boat.

Further complicating matters, I don't have medical insurance right now because while dealing with my kidney stone (and a separate issue involving my gallbladder) I was either working part time or not working at all. As a result, I don't qualify for federal subsidies; any insurance policy would be at least $300 each month, which I can't afford. I would have to meet a deductible before they would start covering appointments and other medical expenses. I'm actually better off not having insurance and paying out of pocket for appointments, especially if I don't need to see doctors frequently. It helps that my urologist, internist, and gastroenterologist give cash patients a 50 percent discount, which is greatly appreciated. Without this, I wouldn't have been able to go as often as I did. However, I know that some other offices require patients to pay the entire amount at the time of your appointment to receive the discount, which isn't always feasible for me. This would mean I'd get billed for the original amount in the future.

For my hospital visits, I didn't have to pay anything upfront, but that was little comfort—I started receiving bills only a couple of weeks after my visits. After discounts, I was still responsible for paying about $4,000, with no reasonable payment plans available. My other three hospital visits were about the same price. Luckily, I was able to get approval to have my visits qualify for charity, which allowed me to cover their costs without paying directly out of pocket. I don't like depending on others for help, but I didn't have much of a choice with three medical bills against my credit already.

If you are in a similar situation, ask your hospital or doctor's office if they offer discounts or charity programs for uninsured or low-income patients. This is something I didn't know about until I received an application in the mail, and I certainly wish I'd known about it much sooner. It would have done a lot to help with the stress I felt over the cost of the health care I needed. I wonder if more people would seek healthcare if they knew about these types of programs.

And I wasn't only worried about paying my immediate medical bills; I was also concerned about paying my monthly bills on time. With decreased work due to illness, I had a decrease in pay, so I had to choose between skipping paying certain bills or asking for help. My parents, who have helped me so much financially, which I'm extremely thankful for, are so wonderful. It is hard for me to continue depending on them for help, but I want everyone reading this to know that it is okay to ask for help financially when it comes to your health care.

8

Awareness

KIDNEY STONES are extremely common, much more so than many people realize. What's more, those who have had one kidney stone in their life are more susceptible to continuing to get them. What this means is that developing kidney stones requires you to change the way you live your life, and that sort of change is never easy. If you have kidney stones, or any other health condition for that matter, you need to know that you are not alone. It's important to have people in your life who support you and care about your well-being. I don't know what I would have done without my family and friends during this trying time.

March is recognized as National Kidney Awareness month, with green being the awareness color for kidney health/kidney illnesses. If you feel comfortable sharing your story of what you've been through, know that it can be very helpful, both for yourself and others, and can allow people to come together in a supportive way. You can also choose to set up events in your community to help educate people about kidney stones and kidney health. By doing so, we send a message to help encourage medical professionals to further research all areas of treatment in hopes of preventing or even curing kidney stones.

Along with the references I have provided, there are many organizations that may be helpful for you to look into. The National Kidney Foundation, the American Association of Kidney Patients, American Kidney Fund, and the Urology Care Association are all great starting points for research and connecting with others. It may also be helpful to look into Facebook groups to connect with others who may be suffering with kidney stones and even the type of kidney stone you have or other kidney issues.

There are different ways you can get involved in kidney stone research and clinical trials if that's something you're interested in participating in. Areas of research that you can participate in at the Mayo Clinic include:

- The efficacy of percutaneous ultrasonic lithotripsy (PUL) after shock wave lithotripsy

- Endoscopic management of upper urinary tract transitional cell carcinoma

- Predicting kidney stone composition using radiographic appearance

- Safely dissolving gallbladder stone fragments using methyl tert-butyl ether immediately after extracorporeal shock wave lithotripsy

- Percutaneous nephrostomy placement as the initial procedure in renal or ureteral calculus removal

- Percutaneous extractions of renal pelvic stones using the Wolf percutaneous universal nephroscopes

The National Institute of Diabetes and Digestive and Kidney Diseases (NIDDK) also conducts research. Open clinical trials can be found at www.ClinicalTrials.gov.

Ask your doctor about your kidney health. There is no such thing as a dumb question, especially when it comes to your own health. If your doctor makes you feel dumb for asking a question, it might be necessary for you to switch doctors. It can be frustrating to essentially start over, but it's critical that you feel like you're being heard and receiving proper care. You're in charge of your health and nobody can take that right from you.

If you know someone who is currently struggling with a kidney stone or other kidney illness, ask them how you can help. Maybe they need someone to buy groceries, run errands, take care of their pet, or cook; maybe they just need someone to listen to what they are going through. Sometimes, we just need someone to let us vent. This is very helpful; I know it goes a long way for me.

Samantha's Experience

Many people don't think about their health until there's a problem; I know I didn't. But by the time I reached the end of my teens, all I could think about was my health. Whenever I had my period and felt awful, it would force me to miss school, work, and planned activities—and it would only get worse from there. I wish we as a society focused more on de-creasing risks of illnesses and symptoms rather than treating ailments after the fact.

Any kind of chronic pain carries with it a risk for developing depression symptoms, and I was no ex-ception. I was depressed, upset, frustrated, and angry at the amount of pain that I was in and I felt like the emergency room and the doctors were refusing to take me seriously. If you feel frustrated in find-ing answers to the point of wanting to give up, I completely understand and I want you to know you aren't alone. I know it's extremely frustrating. Just know that your feelings are valid and that it's okay to talk about them. You are not alone. You are not your illness; you're human and deserve the best possible healthcare, no matter your circumstances. You deserve answers and relief.

I cannot stress enough how important it is that you advocate for yourself when it comes to your health. I hate that it's our responsibility to take charge of our health, even when we're feeling awful and at our worst, but you are the only person that knows how you truly feel. Know that you matter and your health matters. Keep pushing to find the answers you need.

AFTERWORD

THIS BOOK is being published two years after my lithotripsy. I am now working at a local restaurant as an office assistant, which thankfully doesn't require me to stand on my feet for long periods of time—great news for my body. Thankfully, since starting this job, I've only had to call in sick for about three or four days. This is the longest I've been able to work since 2013, and it feels wonderful to be able to support myself and help my family. I'm beyond glad for that.

About halfway through 2020, it did start to feel like I had developed another urinary tract infection; I was extremely nauseous and having problems urinating, as well as right flank pain. I tried taking Azo and drinking cranberry juice, but didn't feel any relief. I thought about going to my local urgent care office because I didn't want to travel two hours one way during the COVID-19 pandemic to see my actual doctor. Ultimately, I decided to go to my out-of-town urologist because he's a great doctor who knows my history and is someone I trust.

My urologist told me that I didn't have a UTI—he didn't see any signs of one—but I did have blood in my urine which suggested...you guessed it, a kidney stone. (It's hard to tell if you have blood in your urine at home unless it's a large amount.) He wrote me a prescription for pain medicine and nausea medicine and we scheduled a follow-up appointment for two weeks later, one which I could do over the phone if I wasn't still experiencing symptoms. He also gave me the option to have a CT scan done that day, or I could wait as a consideration of the amount of radiation involved. He left the decision up to me, which was a big deal. In my experience, many doctors don't do that. Instead, they give you one option and if you don't agree to it they tell you there's nothing they can do for you.

Mindful of the radiation (and grateful for having been given the option to choose), I elected to wait to have a CT scan done. I'd had three done close together between 2018 and 2019 and didn't want to have another one unless I had to. I took the pain medicine and nausea medicine three days in a row due to the amount of pain I was in and my low appetite. A week after my appointment, I felt severely constipated and ended up having to use an enema, because stool softeners weren't helping. After that, I decided not to take the pain medicine and nausea medicine unless I absolutely had to.

The week of my appointment, I decided to call my urologist's office and change my appointment from telehealth to in-person because I was still experiencing pain and didn't feel like I had passed a kidney stone. I also asked if they could schedule a CT scan for me. We did the scan that same day, and I received the results the day after: they showed that I *didn't* have a kidney stone on my right side. This meant I'd either passed it during the two weeks between my first appointment and my CT scan, or I hadn't had one in the first place and it was something else causing my pain. I chose to believe that I'd passed the stone safely, given the presence of blood in my urine at my first appointment.

Reflecting back, if I hadn't gone for a second opinion back in 2019, I probably would have continued having urinary tract infections that may not have been resolved. I still follow the low oxalate diet as much as possible and plan to continue to do so—the pain of kidney stones is one I *never* want to feel again. I truly feel for anyone who has ever had a kidney stone; they're awful and life-changing.

Now looking forward, and thinking about what should be done to improve awareness and treatment of kidney stones, I think it's important that we take a full body approach with our healthcare. All of our body's systems work together to keep us healthy. When one isn't working properly, others can be thrown off and affected, causing problems and long-term damage. For example, nausea is considered a digestive symptom, yet kidney stones affect the urinary system. The brain registers the pain from the kidney stone, while the pain medication I take acts on the neurological system to help decrease pain.

My hope is that doctors will work hard to refer patients to specialists in a timely manner to help them receive proper medical treatment and that more doctors will believe their patients instead of brushing off their pain and symptoms. I also hope that more people will become doctors who specialize so that patients aren't forced to experience long wait times while they are in pain or concerned about their health. And above all, I hope you find some relief if you're suffering with kidney stones.

I'd known for more than a decade that kidney stones run in our family. Given I had almost made it to 30 without a kidney stone, a large part of me hoped that I was finished with health issues. After all, I had already been through my share, hadn't I? Boy, was I wrong. Yet I believe there is a reason for everything. Maybe my reason for having this kidney stone was to write this book, in order to help others with kidney stones and to get a glimpse into what my family has been through over the last decade.

I hope to use my experience with having a kidney stone to help others who are suffering. Whether you've had one kidney stone or ten, you know what that pain feels like; it's certainly not something you'd wish on anyone. Finally, I can't emphasize enough how important it is that we advocate for ourselves and our health. I know sometimes you can't, and I know sometimes it's hard, but it is essential that there be someone in your corner to argue for what you need—and if you're alone in that corner, then that person needs to be you. Just remember that you *deserve* the best health care possible. You *deserve* to be happy, healthy and secure. And you have the right to fight for what you deserve with everything you've got.

RESOURCES AND
RELEVANT RESEARCH

W HEN IT comes to your health, doing your own research plays a huge role in the decision-making process. Learning as much as you can about kidney stones, kidney disease, and other related topics is crucial for your health. In this section, I've provided more research on kidney stones for your reference, including an article published in May 2020 by the Children's Hospital of Philadelphia which discusses how a world-renowned pediatric kidney stone expert is using past research to explore how changes in the gut microbiome influence kidney stone formation.

Kidney stone surgeries have come a long way, and can now be done in a minimally invasive fashion which usually doesn't require incisions. This, too, is due to research and medical innovation. This makes it easier for patients to heal, hopefully increasing a patient's quality of life.

According to Urology Austin, "Kidney disease is the ninth leading cause of death in the United States".[14] Our kidneys "work hard in maintaining overall health by filtering waste and regulating salt, potassium, and acid".[14] The kidneys are "organs [that] produce an active form of Vitamin D that promotes healthy bones". Does this mean that patients who have a low blood level of Vitamin D (25-Hydroxy Vitamin D) are more susceptible to kidney stones?

The kidneys help the body use Vitamin D by converting its raw form into the active form, which is what is used by the body. Without an adequate intake of Vitamin D , the body could suffer from problems like osteoporosis, heart disease, depression, and rickets. It's important that we talk to our doctors about having our Vitamin D levels checked and know what our levels are so we can start treatment if needed.

In the 1970s, the prevalence of a kidney stone was 3.8%, whereas in the 2000s it's been about 8.8%.[1] This is a huge increase, so what's changed? Is it related to genetics and we are just finding out about it? Is it related to diet? Also, people who have one kidney stone in their lifetime are at a higher risk to develop more stones in their future.[1] The Urology Care Association states that 1 out of every 3 (33%) of Americans are at risk of kidney disease. This organization also estimates that one out of every 10 Americans will have kidney stones at some point in their lifetime.[15] Kidney stones are considered the most common disease of the urinary system.

Factors that can put people at a higher risk of kidney disease include diabetes, high blood pressure, and a family history of kidney problems. Blood and urine tests can be done at your doctor's office to determine how your kidneys are functioning

A kidney stone is not the same as kidney disease and risk does not mean that you have the ailment. However, I think it's important to make others aware of this so they can be proactive in their health and know what to look out for.

The Rare Diseases Clinical Research Network's website lists ways people can be involved in different research studies for different rare illnesses associated with kidney stone formation.[16] The rare disorders that are being studied include: primary hyperoxaluria (PH), enteric hyperoxuria (EH), cystinuria, adenine phosphoribosyltransferase (APRT) deficiency, and Dent disease.

According to an article published by *Advances in Urology*, calcium oxalate kidney stones are formed in the part of the kidney called Randall's plaque, which is on the kidney papillary surface. This article discusses how "kidney stones have been associated with an increased risk of chronic kidney diseases, end-stage renal failure, cardiovascular diseases, diabetes, and hypertension".[17] These kidney health concerns are all serious health issues. This is why kidney stones need to be treated as soon as possible and why it's important to make the necessary diet and lifestyle changes.

According to *Reviews in Urology*, diverticulum, also called "calyceal diverticula are rare outpouchings of the upper collecting system that likely have a congenital origin".[18] Congenital, meaning someone who has any number of diverticulum, was born with them and they may cause problems at any point in life. Just because someone is born with something, doesn't mean that they'll show signs or symptoms of it immediately. Problems occur when kidney stones are found in these outpouchings because they have no way to get out without some type of intervention. Kidney stones cause infections and they need to be removed as soon as possible so they don't cause more chronic problems down the road. Kidney stones "can be found in up to 50% of cases [with diverticula], the vast majority of patients are asymptomatic and chronic pain, recurrent urinary tract infection, gross hematuria, or decline in renal function" are reasons to operate on diverticulum.[18] Laparoscopic surgery may be necessary and involves minimally invasive incisions for the surgeon to decide how to proceed with the patient's treatment and healthcare. If you have recurrent kidney infections and stones, it may be beneficial to talk to your doctor about the possibility of diverticulum, which treatment options and operations they feel comfortable with providing, and the best way for you to move forward in your health care.

An article published by *Advanced Urology* discusses kidney stone disease. It is "a crystal concretion found usually in the kidneys".[19] Kidney stones are like sand, concrete, or pebbles depending on their size. These numbers are increasing and is said to affect about 12 percent of the human population. Kidney stone disease can be associated with end-stage renal failure, which is scary to say the least. Our kidneys are so important to our daily function and overall health even though we may not think about it until we run into an issue.

APPENDIX A:
WHAT TO BRING TO A
DOCTOR'S APPOINTMENT

If you've ever been bounced around from doctor to doctor, you know how crucial it is to keep good records—what you've been tested for, what treatments you've tried, which surgeries you've had (or refused to have), as well as any other helpful information.

The following is an example of what you could take with you to a doctor's appointment, especially to a first visit with a new practitioner, to ensure that any doctor you meet with has a full understanding of (and appreciation for) what you've already been through. (While not included here, it may also be helpful to include the doctor's name and their specialty alongside the treatment options they prescribed.)

It is also extremely important to keep copies of all of your medical records to have on hand at any given time. I know this may seem like an overwhelming and daunting task, but it will be extremely beneficial for you in the long run.

Medical Timeline

Medications Tried for Kidney Stone and Urinary Symptoms

- Toradol

- Flomax

- AZO

- Keflex

- Pyridium

- Bactrim

- Aleve/Naproxen

- Norco

Diagnoses

- Endometriosis

- Polycystic Ovary Syndrome (PCOS)

- Interstitial Cystitis (IC)

- Vitamin D Deficiency

- Retroperitoneal Fibrosis

- Osteoporosis

- Irritable Bowel Syndrome (IBS)

- Minimum Mitral Valve Prolapse

- History of kidney stone

- High liver enzymes

Surgeries/Procedures

- Tonsils and adenoids removed: 1996

- Tubes in and out of ears: 1996

- Multiple CT scans, MRIs, and ultrasounds since 2009

- Laparoscopic surgery for endometriosis: 2010, 2012, 2013, 2014, 2015, 2016

- Colonoscopy: 2011, 2016

- Appendix removed: 2013

- Complete hysterectomy (both ovaries, uterus, and cervix removed): 2014

- Gallbladder removed: 2016

- Left knee arthroscope: 2017

- Lithotripsy: January 2019

- Last CT scan: February 2019

APPENDIX B:
WHAT TO ASK
YOUR DOCTOR

No matter how many times you go to a doctor's office, it never stops being overwhelming. That's why it can be helpful to bring a list of general and specific questions with you to make sure that you get all the information you need.

The following is a sample list of basic questions I find helpful to ask any new doctor I see, as well as some specific to kidney stone related issues:

- I'm having flank pain. What tests can be done to determine if I have a kidney stone or some other kidney illness?

- What type of kidney stone do I have?

- What treatment options do I have for a kidney stone and to help with the pain?

- Are there side effects to any of the treatments you're recommending?

- Will these treatments place me at a higher risk for other illnesses?

- Do you work with other doctors or can you refer patients to specialists for treatment?

- If you are unsure how to treat my illness, can you refer me to a specialist?

- Do you test for other illnesses if needed? If not, can you refer me to a doctor or specialist who performs the necessary testing?

ABOUT THE AUTHOR

S AMANTHA BOWICK has a Master of Public Health (MPH) degree from Liberty University. She received her Bachelor of Science degree in Health Care Administration at Columbia Southern University. She is devoted to using her education and experiences to advocate for people who suffer with chronic illnesses through her organization Chronic Illness Support, LLC. If you would like to connect with Samantha further, you can find her on her Website (https::// www.samanthabowick.com), Facebook (Samantha Bowick or Chronic Illness Support, LLC) Twitter (@skbowick), and Instagram (@skbowick).

D R. DAVID BRANDLI received his Bachelor of Science degree in Kinesiology from UCLA in 1990 and continued his education at Jefferson Medical College with a master's degree in molecular biology. He received his medical degree from Penn State University and completed residency training in General Surgery and Urology at Indiana University in Indianapolis. He has been board certified in urology since 2005. Although he practices general urology, he has special interests in oncology and kidney stone disease. Throughout his career, he has published more than 20 scientific abstracts and peer-reviewed journal articles and given scientific presentations and lectures on various topics in urology. Dr. Brandli was voted second in the 2017 Best Urologists by Mount Pleasant Magazine. He is active in several clinical committees in area hospitals, and is a member of the American Urologic Association, the American Association of Clinical Urologists, the America Endourologic Association, and the American Society of Laparoscopic Surgeons.

REFERENCES

1 https://www.kidney.org/atoz/content/kidneystones

2 https://ghr.nlm.nih.gov/condition/kidney-stones

3 https://nyulangone.org/conditions/kidney-stones-in-adults/types

4 https://www.kidney.org/atoz/content/kidneystones

5 https://www.kidney.org/atoz/content/kidneystones_shockwave

6 https://www.kidney.org/atoz/content/kidneystones_shockwave

7 https://www.ncbi.nlm.nih.gov/pmc/articles/PMC4004282/

8 https://www.nccih.nih.gov/health/probiotics-what-you-need-to-know

9 https://www.health.harvard.edu/blog/what-causes-kidney-stones-and-what-to-do-2019051716656.

10 http://www.pkdiet.com/pdf/LowOxalateDiet.pdf

11 https://www.thevpfoundation.org/index.htm

12 https://northaustinurology.com/resources/low-oxalate-diet/

13 https://www.niddk.nih.gov/health-information/urologic-diseases/kidney-stones/eating-diet-nutrition

[14] https://urologyaustin.com/march-national-kidney-awareness-month-kidney-stones/

[15] http://urologyhealth.org/careblog/march-is-national-kidney-month-x3078

[16] https://www.rarediseasesnetwork.org/cms/rksc/Get-Involved/Studies/6401

[17] https://www.ncbi.nlm.nih.gov/pmc/articles/PMC5817324/

[18] https://www.ncbi.nlm.nih.gov/pmc/articles/PMC4004282/

[19] https://www.ncbi.nlm.nih.gov/pmc/articles/PMC5817324/

ALSO BY SAMANTHA BOWICK

Living with Endometriosis

Living with Alpha-1 Antitrypsin Deficiency

Living with Endometriosis Workbook and Daily Journal

My Health Journal

_____

_____

_____

_____

_____

_____

_____

_____

_____

_____

_____

_____

_____

_____

_____

_____

_____

_____

My Health Journal

_____

_____

_____

_____

_____

_____

_____

_____

_____

_____

_____

_____

_____

_____

_____

_____

_____

_____

My Health Journal

My Health Journal

_____

_____

_____

_____

_____

_____

_____

_____

_____

_____

_____

_____

_____

_____

_____

_____

_____

_____

My Health Journal

_____

_____

_____

_____

_____

_____

_____

_____

_____

_____

_____

_____

_____

_____

_____

_____

My Health Journal

_____

_____

_____

_____

_____

_____

_____

_____

_____

_____

_____

_____

_____

_____

_____

_____

_____

_____

_____

My Health Journal

_____

_____

_____

_____

_____

_____

_____

_____

_____

_____

_____

_____

_____

_____

_____

_____

_____